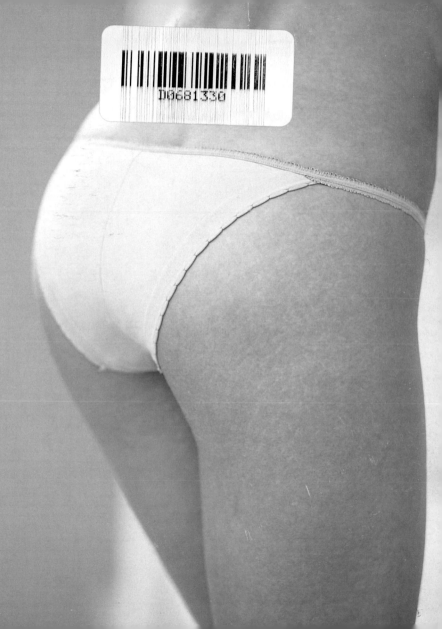

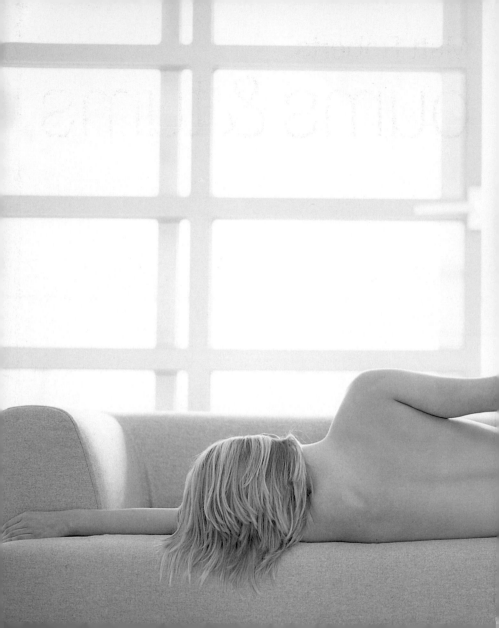

Matt Roberts
bums & tums

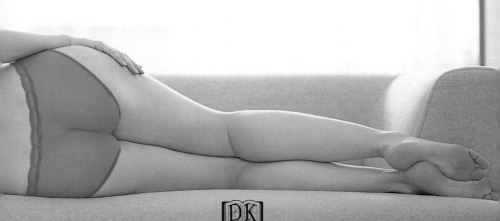

DK

A Dorling Kindersley Book

LONDON, NEW YORK, MUNICH,
MELBOURNE, and DELHI

This book is for my wife Helen

Editors Michael Fullalove, Anna Fischel

Project Art Editor Janis Utton

Managing Editor Gillian Roberts

Category Publisher Mary-Clare Jerram

Art Director Tracy Killick

DTP Designer Sonia Charbonnier

Production Controller Louise Daly

Photographer Russell Sadur

First published in Great Britain in 2003
by Dorling Kindersley Limited
80 Strand, London WC2R 0RL
A Penguin Company

Copyright © 2003 Dorling Kindersley Limited, London

Text Copyright © 2003 Matt Roberts Personal Training

4 6 8 10 9 7 5 3

Always consult your doctor before starting a fitness and/or nutrition
programme if you have any health concerns.

A CIP catalogue record for this book is available from
The British Library

ISBN 0 7513 4877 5

Colour reproduced by GRB, Italy

Printed and bound by Printer Trento, Italy

See our complete catalogue at www.dk.com

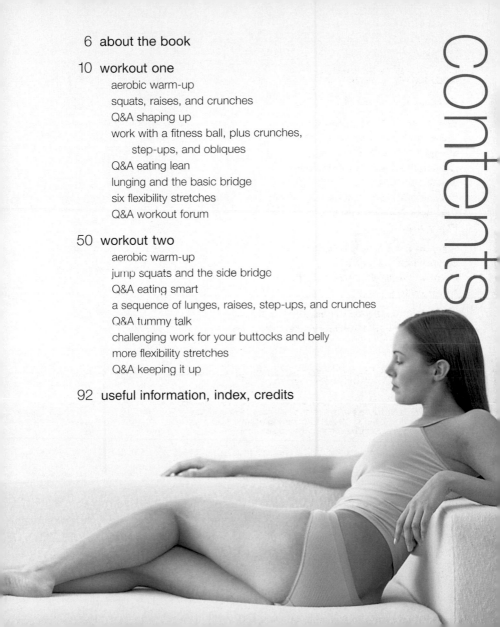

contents

6 about the book

10 workout one
    aerobic warm-up
    squats, raises, and crunches
    Q&A shaping up
    work with a fitness ball, plus crunches,
        step-ups, and obliques
    Q&A eating lean
    lunging and the basic bridge
    six flexibility stretches
    Q&A workout forum

50 workout two
    aerobic warm-up
    jump squats and the side bridge
    Q&A eating smart
    a sequence of lunges, raises, step-ups, and crunches
    Q&A tummy talk
    challenging work for your buttocks and belly
    more flexibility stretches
    Q&A keeping it up

92 useful information, index, credits

about the book

If you had the choice between a visit to a plastic surgeon and a consultation with a personal trainer, I wonder which you'd choose. Much would depend on what you were after, of course: no end of step-ups is ever going to give you a ski-jump nose. But if it was a beautiful bottom and a flat tummy you wanted, then there's actually no contest: go for the trainer every time. Why? Well, as a friend of mine who's a plastic surgeon himself always says, "there are changes you can make to your body shape with exercise that the knife simply can't achieve". And to prove it, he sends a steady stream of clients to my gym.

Bums and tums are perennial problem areas. They're the features women complain about most. They're where the body stores fat naturally, and where it's hardest to shift. But flattening your tummy and shaping your bottom needn't be hell. With the correct combination of exercise and nutrition, you can turn a tired and slack behind into a pert and peachy posterior; and if your waist's gone AWOL, you can bring it right back into line.

I've devised two workouts of simple exercises for you, with the emphasis bang on those two areas. To do them, you

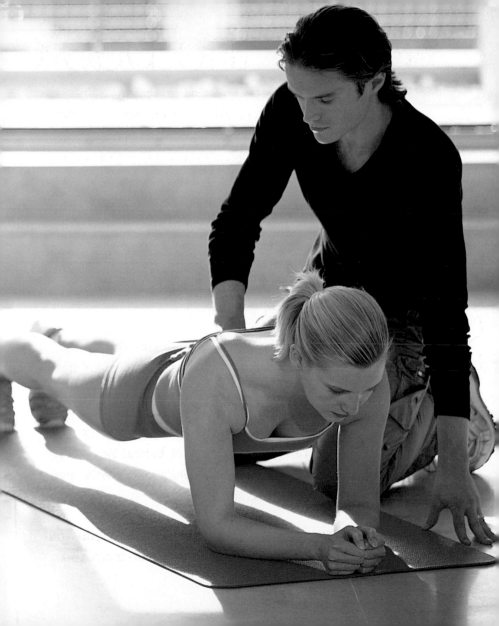

don't have to set foot in a gym and you don't need tons of fancy equipment. You can do them at home with just a fitness ball. To maximize their effectiveness, I've given the workouts a combined approach. There are dynamic moves like crunches and curls to blitz your belly. Other exercises target particular muscles – those at the side of your waist, say. To burn fat and sculpt your buttocks, there are short bursts of aerobic activity. I've also included some stretches to keep your muscles long and lean. And, because I know there's more to getting a pert bottom and a trim waist than exercise alone, I'll be passing on the answers to those questions my clients ask me most, advising you on your technique, and giving you tips about topics like healthy eating, detox, and cellulite.

So, come on. Set aside 30 minutes every other day. Stick to my workouts. And the bum and the tum of your dreams can be yours in just a matter of weeks.

Here's to the new you!

Matt

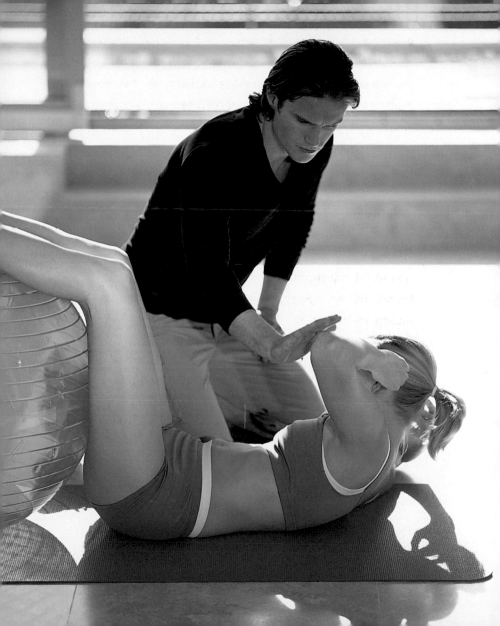

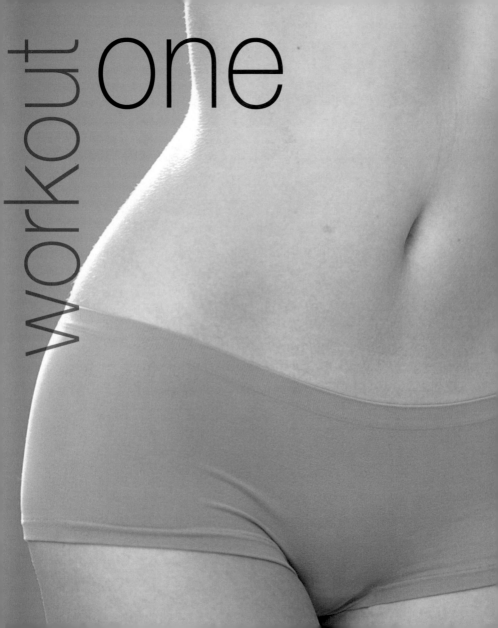

workout one

Get set for the fat-burning and muscle-sculpting. The blitz on your buttocks, stomach, and hips starts right here. You're about to become leaner, stronger, sexier, and undeniably more toned.

aerobic warm-up

Before you start the exercises in workout one, you need to warm up for 5–10 minutes to prepare your muscles. Power walking or running are the ideal choices because they burn fat and tone muscle. Do whichever feels most comfortable. Here are some tips for your technique.

● When power walking, make sure that as you're stepping forwards you plant your heel first, then roll through with your body weight. At the same time, bring your front hand up to about chest height (but don't bring it too high).

● When your weight is on your front foot, push your back leg into the stride (you should feel your buttocks and thighs working). Pull your other arm back strongly as you do so.

Running requires more power than walking. It's also high impact, so wear good trainers. And make sure you:

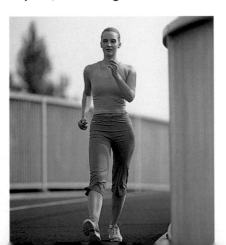

● Take short fast strides.
● Avoid high knee-lifts and big bouncy steps (these will only tire you and strain your joints).

Once you've warmed up, move straight on to the seated squat.

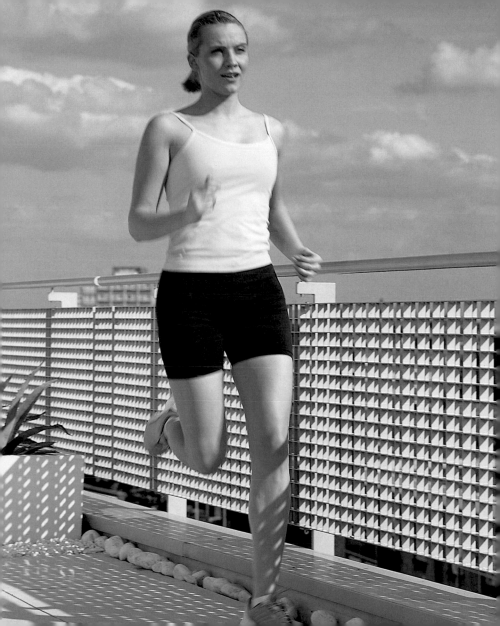

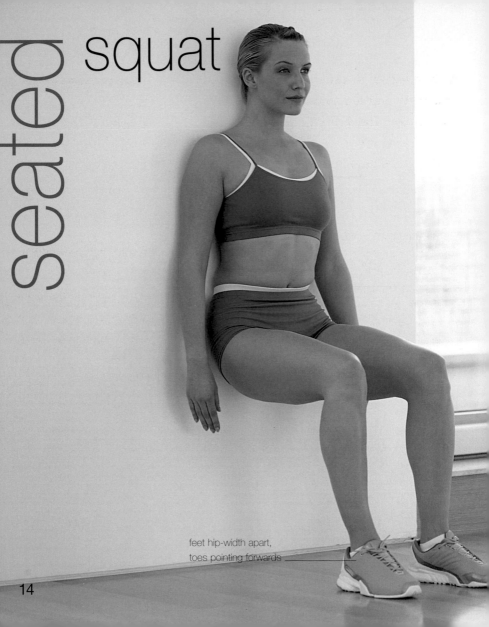

seated squat

feet hip-width apart,
toes pointing forwards

**A bit of a killer to start with, so grit
your teeth and remember to keep your
body weight towards your heels.**

level ①* hold the position for 30 secs
level ②* hold the position for 60 secs

Stand with your back flat against a wall and
your feet about 30cm (12in) from it. Keep
your arms relaxed by your sides. Slowly
slide your body down the wall until your
thighs are parallel with the floor. Adjust
your foot position so your lower legs are
completely upright, then pull your belly in
towards your spine and hold the position
still for the required time.

do it right

rests between exercises

Get into the habit of resting for
up to 30 seconds between
exercises. These mini-breaks
are ideal moments to have a sip
of water – remember your body
dehydrates during exercise.

breathing correctly

One other thing to keep an eye
on is your breathing. Practise
breathing in before you move
and out as you move. Keep
your tummy muscles taut and
pulled in all the time. Above all,
don't hold your breath!

* check your level on p92

glute raise

This exercise 'lifts' your bottom by concentrating the work on the upper part of it. Make sure you keep your hips pinned to the floor to stop yourself rolling around.

level ① do 20 raises per leg

level ② do 30 raises per leg

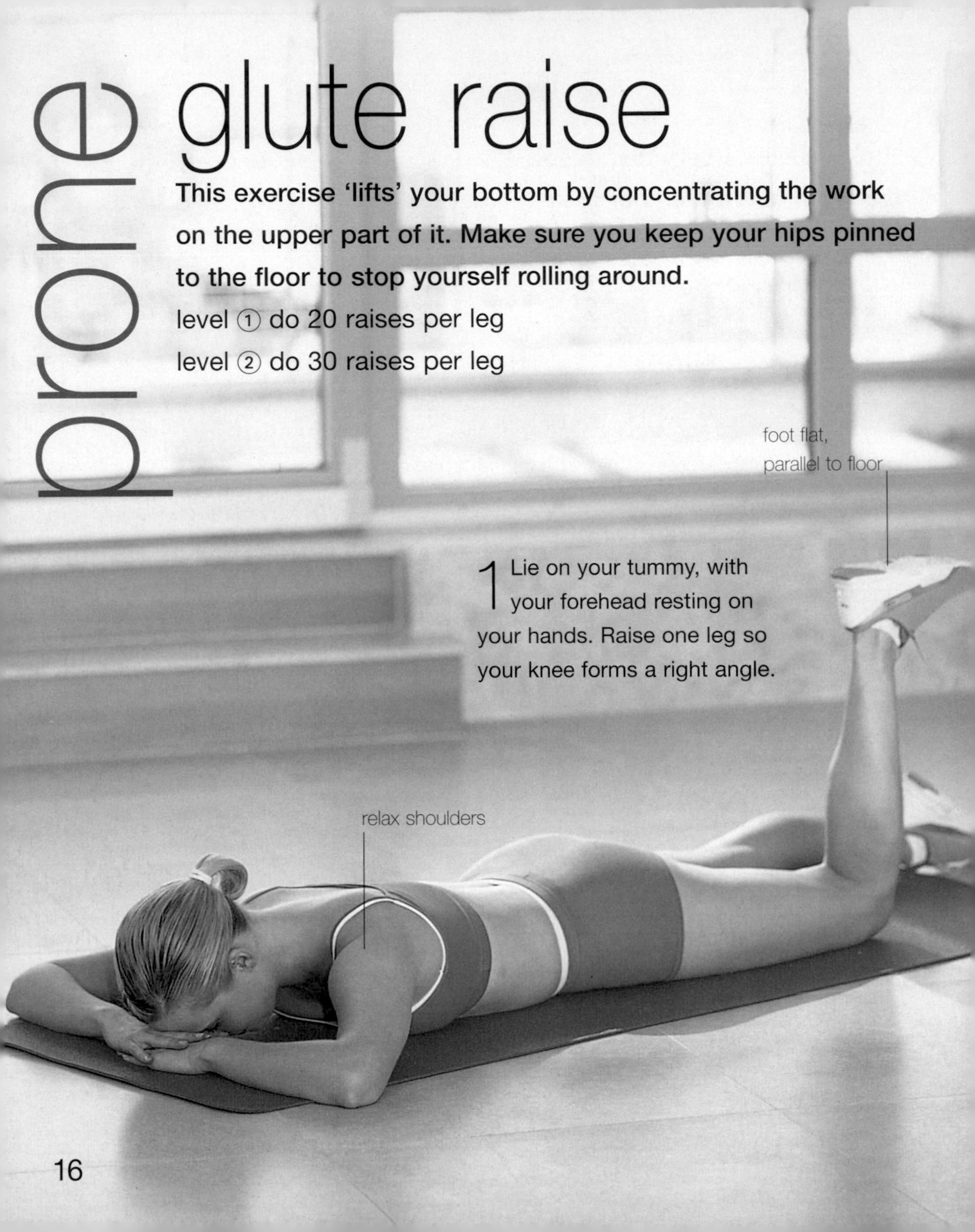

foot flat, parallel to floor

1 Lie on your tummy, with your forehead resting on your hands. Raise one leg so your knee forms a right angle.

relax shoulders

2 Squeezing your buttocks, and pushing the sole of your foot up towards the ceiling, lift your leg up as high as feels comfortable. Slowly lower your leg to the start position. Keep your hips flat on the floor throughout. When you've done all the raises with one leg, switch legs and repeat.

keep hips still

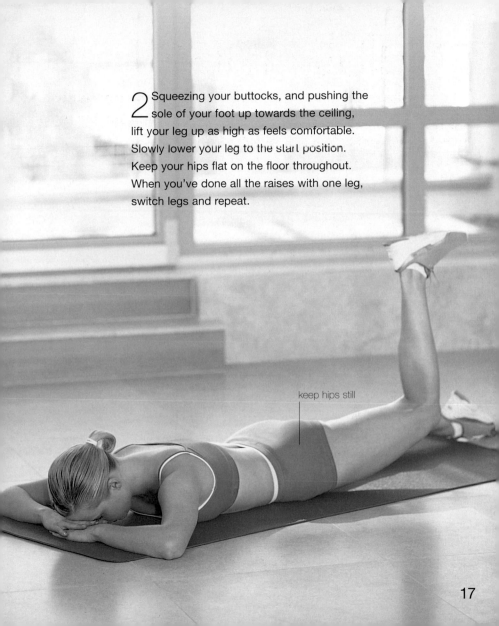

full crunch

This exercise looks simple enough, but it's actually quite tricky. To get it right, you need balance and coordination.

level ① do 15 crunches

level ② do 30 crunches

1 Lie on your back with your legs in the air, your knees bent, and your hands by your ears.

keep your back flat, don't arch it

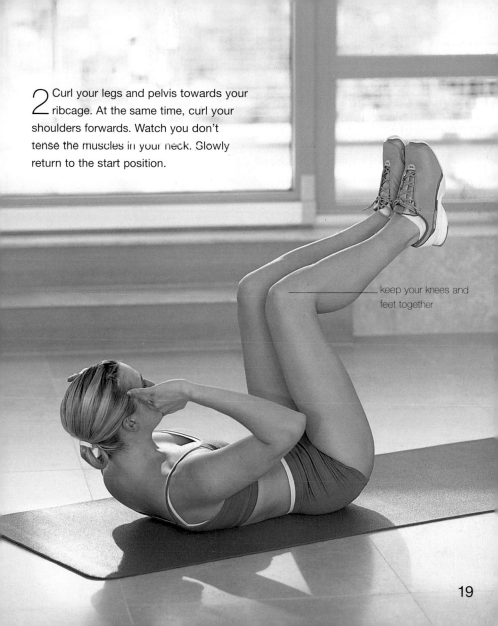

2 Curl your legs and pelvis towards your
ribcage. At the same time, curl your
shoulders forwards. Watch you don't
tense the muscles in your neck. Slowly
return to the start position.

keep your knees and
feet together

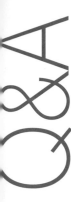

shaping up

How can I make my buttocks more pert and round?

It's best to do it with some kind of 'resistance work'. The exercises in this book count as resistance work because you're using your body weight as resistance, but you could equally do exercises that call for free weights, for example. The muscles in your buttocks respond well to a stimulus of this kind, so you should be able to shape them up in no time. If your figure's verging on the pear-shaped, you may need to count the calories for a while as well, and burn fat with some aerobic work such as running – three or four sessions of about 30 minutes per week should do it.

What exercises can I do to narrow my waist?

Any exercise that works your stomach muscles or your obliques (the muscles at the side of your waist) is ideal, as are exercises that target your lower back. Crunches and curls are particularly good waist exercises to concentrate on, and are more fun with a fitness ball. The side bridge too is a superb waist-toner. Do bear in mind, however, that genetics play a large part in how small your waist will become.

Will these workouts improve my 'core strength'?

Core strength's a real buzz word right now. It refers to the band of muscles that runs round your midriff like a wide belt from waist to hip. All the exercises in these workouts will improve your core strength and give you a flatter stomach, better posture, and a firmer, problem-free back.

I'd love to be able to wear jeans but I always feel so self-conscious because of the roll of fat that sticks out around the waistband. What can I do about it?

To get rid of your 'spare tyre', you need to start burning more calories than you take in. Rather than simply eating less, try changing what you eat. Fill up on fruit and veg so that you're not snacking on high-calorie, nutrient-poor fast foods. Combine this healthy eating with at least 30 minutes aerobic exercise three or four times a week. And stick to the workouts – you'll soon look fantastic in jeans.

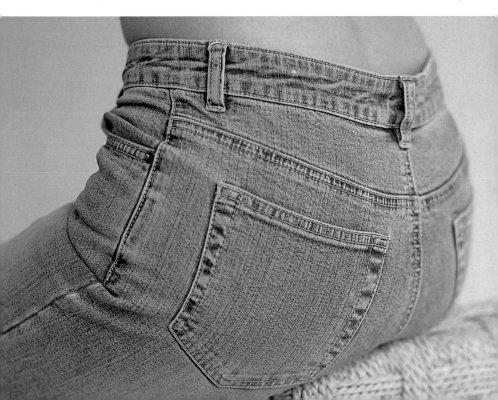

curl with ball

The best exercise outside of the gym for the backs of your thighs. To make it even more effective, raise your hips off the floor in step 1 and then keep them raised.

level ① do 20 curls

level ② do 30 curls

1 Place the fitness ball against a wall. Lie on your back with your arms by your sides and your palms to the floor. Rest your feet on the middle of the ball. Keep your heels knee-width apart and your toes pointing up.

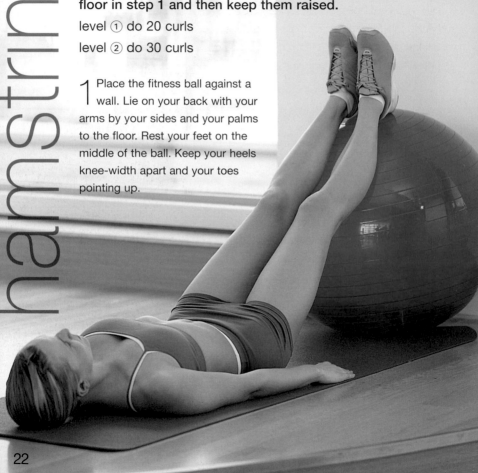

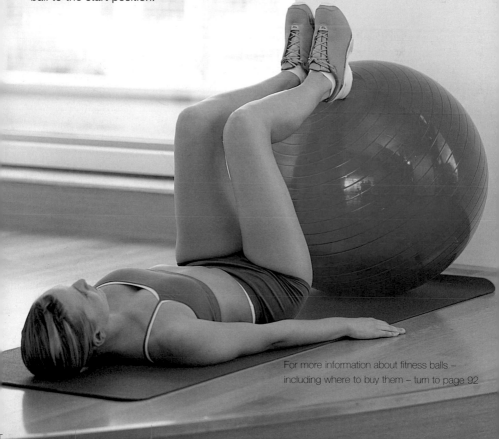

2 Gently push your heels in to the top of the ball, then pull them slowly towards you, dragging the ball about 20cm (8in) towards you as you do so. Keep your head, shoulders, and arms still. Slowly return your legs and the ball to the start position.

For more information about fitness balls – including where to buy them – turn to page 92

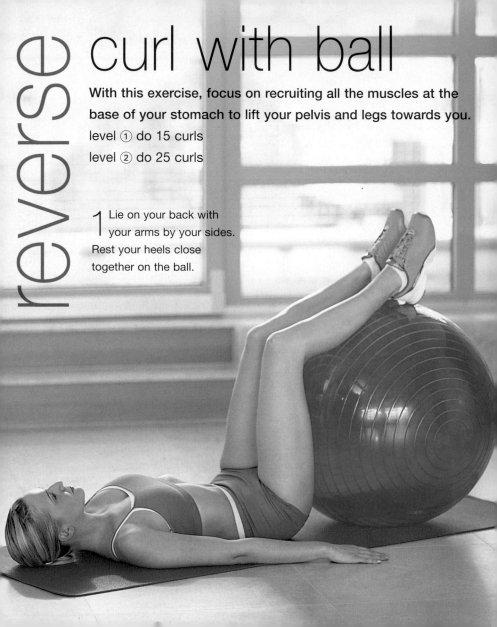

reverse curl with ball

With this exercise, focus on recruiting all the muscles at the base of your stomach to lift your pelvis and legs towards you.

level ① do 15 curls

level ② do 25 curls

1 Lie on your back with your arms by your sides. Rest your heels close together on the ball.

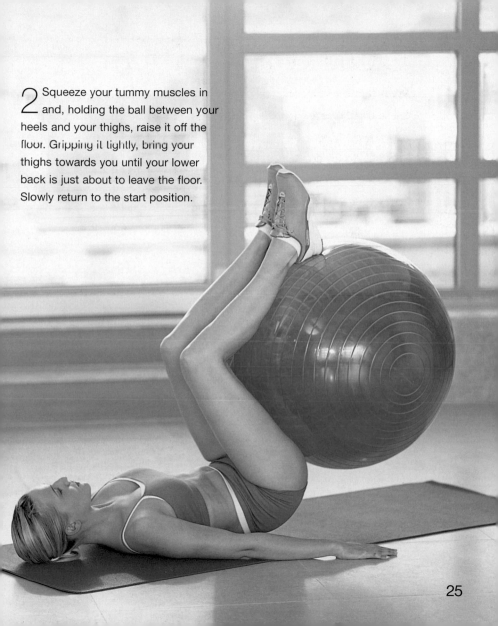

2 Squeeze your tummy muscles in and, holding the ball between your heels and your thighs, raise it off the floor. Gripping it lightly, bring your thighs towards you until your lower back is just about to leave the floor. Slowly return to the start position.

raise on ball

Part of the reason this exercise is so effective is that it calls for good balance and control. Feel the work in your buttocks and at the backs of your thighs. And keep your back straight.

level ① do 15 raises

level ② do 25 raises

1 Lie on your back with your legs together and your feet and calves on the ball. Rest your arms by your sides, palms to the floor.

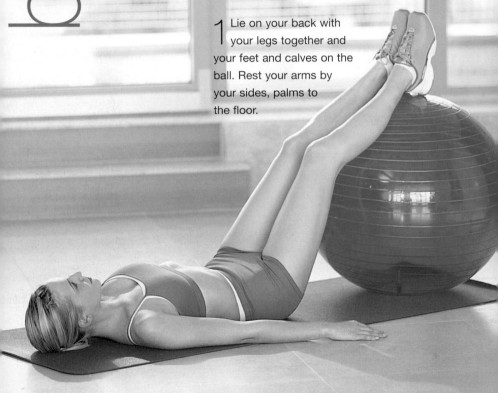

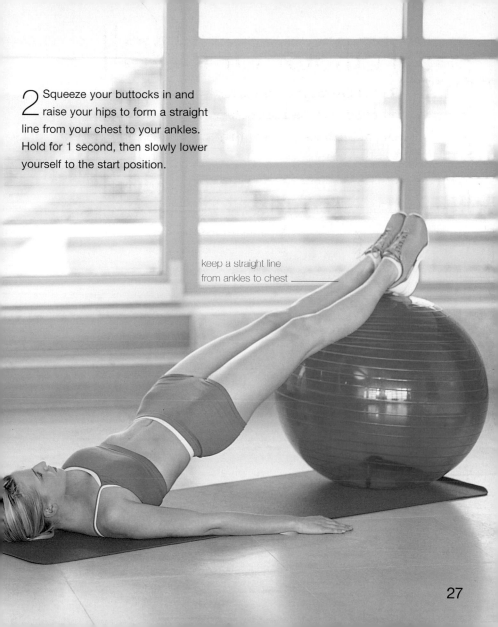

2 Squeeze your buttocks in and
raise your hips to form a straight
line from your chest to your ankles.
Hold for 1 second, then slowly lower
yourself to the start position.

keep a straight line
from ankles to chest _____

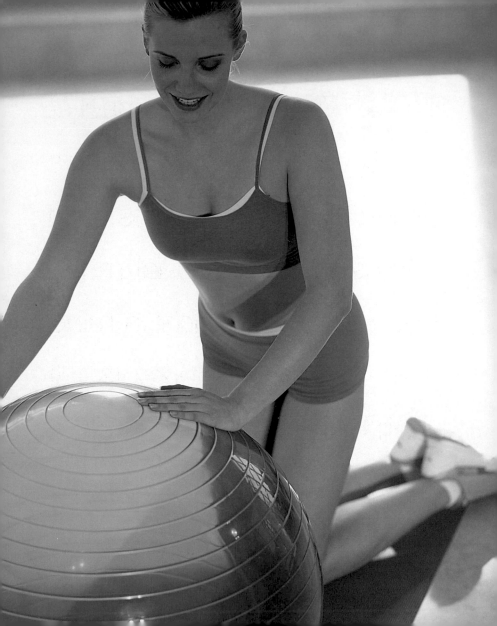

When your stomach's tighter and your bottom's firmer, your jeans, skirts, and trousers will all fit that much better. Keep this goal in mind as you do the workouts – it will help you put in the hard work you need to do.

leg crunch

The difference between this and a regular crunch is small, but your raised leg places pressure on your obliques (the muscles at the side of your waist) and your abdominals from a different angle. The result? A well-corseted waist.

level ① do 15 crunches per leg

level ② do 25 crunches per leg

1 Lie flat on your back with one foot on the ground and the other leg raised in front of you. Get your thighs parallel. Place your hands by your ears.

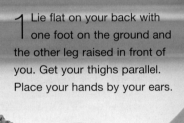

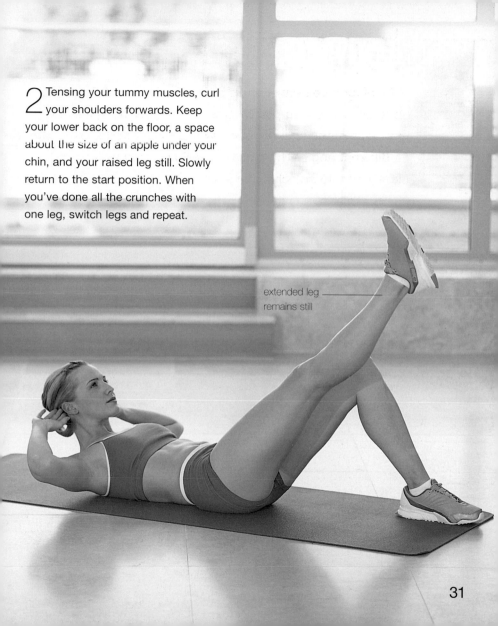

2 Tensing your tummy muscles, curl your shoulders forwards. Keep your lower back on the floor, a space about the size of an apple under your chin, and your raised leg still. Slowly return to the start position. When you've done all the crunches with one leg, switch legs and repeat.

extended leg remains still

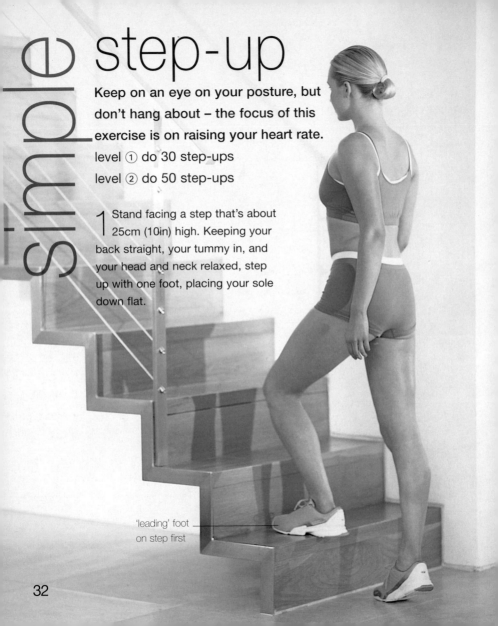

simple step-up

Keep on an eye on your posture, but don't hang about – the focus of this exercise is on raising your heart rate.

level ① do 30 step-ups

level ② do 50 step-ups

1 Stand facing a step that's about 25cm (10in) high. Keeping your back straight, your tummy in, and your head and neck relaxed, step up with one foot, placing your sole down flat.

'leading' foot ⎯⎯⎯⎯ on step first

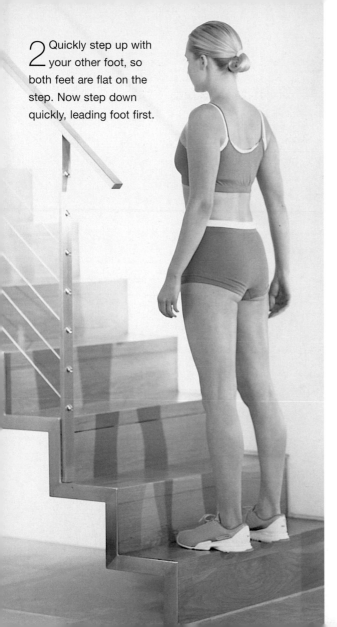

2 Quickly step up with your other foot, so both feet are flat on the step. Now step down quickly, leading foot first.

variation

for next time

The next time you do the step-up, 'lead' with your other foot. After that, switch leading foot with every workout.

make it harder

If you'd like a more difficult version of the step-up, try the knee raise. It's tough, but works as many of your leg muscles in as many directions as possible. Perform step 1 as horo. In step 2, rather than placing your foot on the step, raise your knee straight to hip height. Lower your knee and place your foot back on the floor. Step down with your other foot, then do the next knee raise with your other leg. Continue alternating legs.

oblique

Resting your legs on the ball in this exercise makes you work your waist muscles harder as you rotate your body.

level ① do 15 obliques per side

level ② do 25 obliques per side

1 Lie flat on your back, with your heels and calves resting close together on the ball. Make sure you tuck the ball in tight against your thighs. Place your hands by your ears.

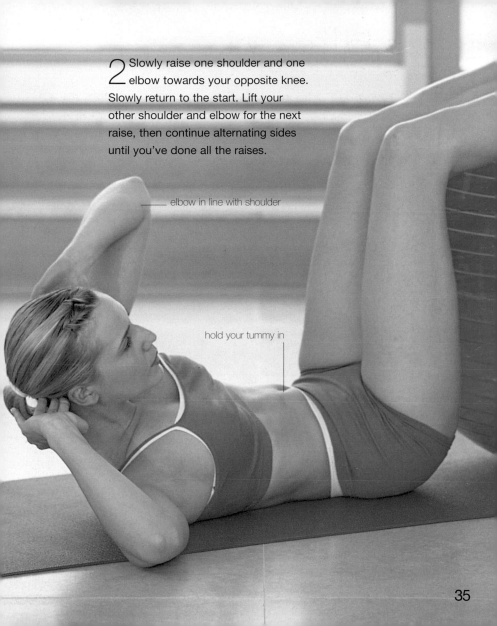

2 Slowly raise one shoulder and one elbow towards your opposite knee. Slowly return to the start. Lift your other shoulder and elbow for the next raise, then continue alternating sides until you've done all the raises.

_____ elbow in line with shoulder

hold your tummy in

eating lean

I feel bloated after meals even though I don't eat that much. A friend of mine was telling me about her wheat intolerance recently and I wonder if that could be my problem too. What do you think?

Even if you're not actually intolerant to wheat, you could simply be eating too much of it. It's easily done – cereal for breakfast, sandwich for lunch, pasta for dinner – and the effect can be bloating. Try cutting down so you have wheat only once a day. In its place, eat oat-based cereals and grains such as quinoa, millet, brown rice, and wild rice. And when you do eat wheat, have it in a fairly unrefined form, so the pasta you eat should be wholewheat and the bread wholemeal.

What slimming diet do you recommend?

In short, none. There's mounting evidence that weight-reducing diets don't work, even if there's an initial loss. A dramatic cut in calories puts your body in starvation mode and reduces your metabolic rate. So when you eat normally again, your body doesn't use all the calories, but stores the unused fuel as fat. Do your best to stick to the workouts, and make your diet healthy. I aim to eat little and often, and as healthily as I can without getting obsessed. Set a target of two healthy meals out of three, and make the bulk of them vegetables and fruit. Don't worry about the odd bar of chocolate or glass of wine either. You'll look and feel ten times better for the occasional treat.

I don't seem to be able to stop myself nibbling. Why?

It may be that your blood sugar levels are fluctuating too widely. When you eat foods that fuel your body rapidly with 'sugar', your body quickly wants more, urging you on to nibble. Many of the staples of western diets – like potatoes, cereals, and sugary foods – fall into this category. Foods that drip-feed your body with 'sugar', on the other hand, bypass these energy peaks and troughs. They include most kinds of fruit and vegetable, beans and lentils, white fish, chicken, and turkey. Make the most of them.

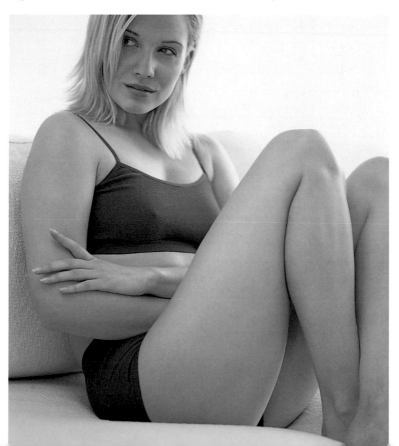

simple lunge

One of my favourites. It's nice and simple, but it works your legs hard. Keep a close eye on your posture.

level ① do 15 lunges per leg

level ② do 25 lunges per leg

1 Place one foot in front of you about one stride-length from your back foot. Keep your hips facing forward and your hands relaxed by your sides. Stand up straight and pull your tummy muscles in.

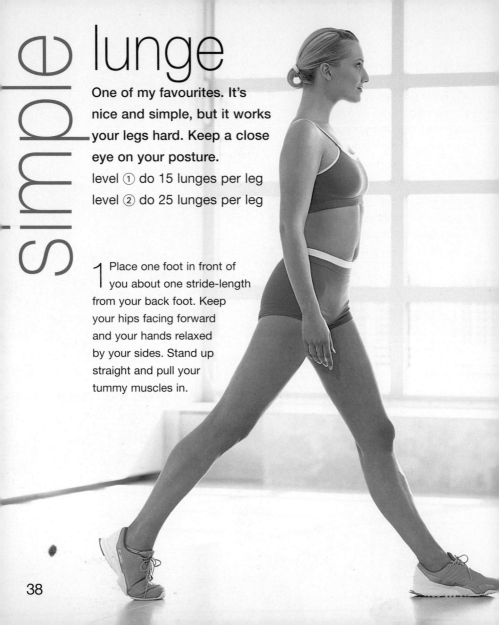

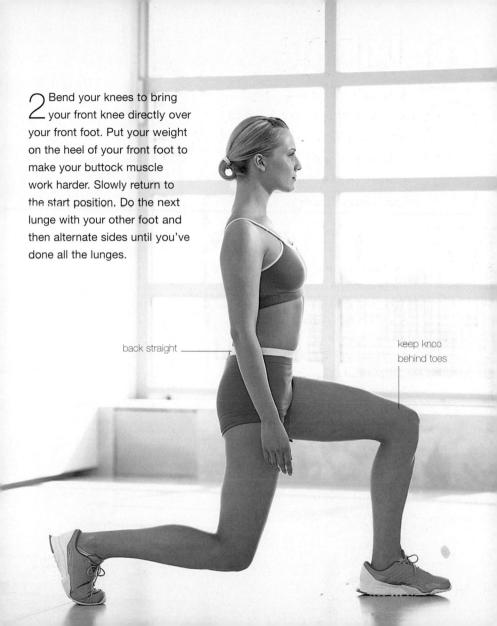

2 Bend your knees to bring your front knee directly over your front foot. Put your weight on the heel of your front foot to make your buttock muscle work harder. Slowly return to the start position. Do the next lunge with your other foot and then alternate sides until you've done all the lunges.

back straight

keep knee behind toes

basic bridge

To prove that you don't always need to move to work effectively, this 'hold' uses all the muscles in your torso, and uses them hard.

level ① hold for 30 secs

level ② hold for 60 secs

1 Position yourself with your toes on the floor and your elbows directly under your shoulders.

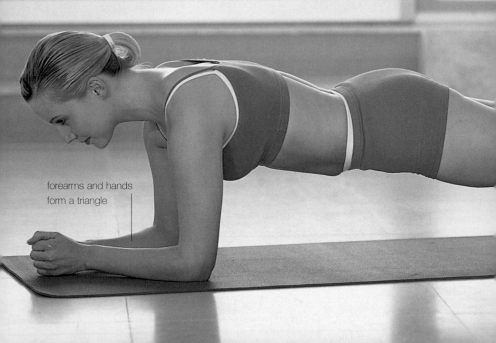

forearms and hands form a triangle

2 Keeping a straight line from your shoulders to your ankles, raise yourself up so your elbows and toes support your body. Use your tummy muscles to maintain the position, and watch you don't stick your bottom in the air. Slowly return to the start.

now repeat the workout

When you've performed the bridge, go back to page 14 and do all the exercises again in order. After you've done the bridge for a second time, finish your workout with the stretch moves overleaf.

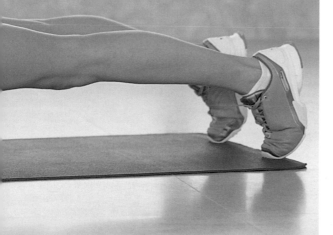

body talk

solving cellulite

One topic I'm often asked about is cellulite – the layer of orange-peel-like fat that appears on bottoms, thighs, and arms. Cellulite picks its victims indiscriminately – you certainly don't need a lot of body fat to suffer from it. But what does cause it? And what can you do about it?

- Cellulite is the result of a build-up of toxins in fat cells.
- To help combat it, take regular exercise (the sort you're doing now) and have the occasional massage.
- Follow a programme of detox to 'cleanse' the fat cells: cut out alcohol, tea, and coffee, and replace them with water, fruit juice, and fruit teas.

You're almost at the end of workout one now – only some stretching to go. The exercises you've just done have worked as many of your muscle groups as possible whenever possible. Which is why you're bang on line for a stronger, leaner-looking bum and tum.

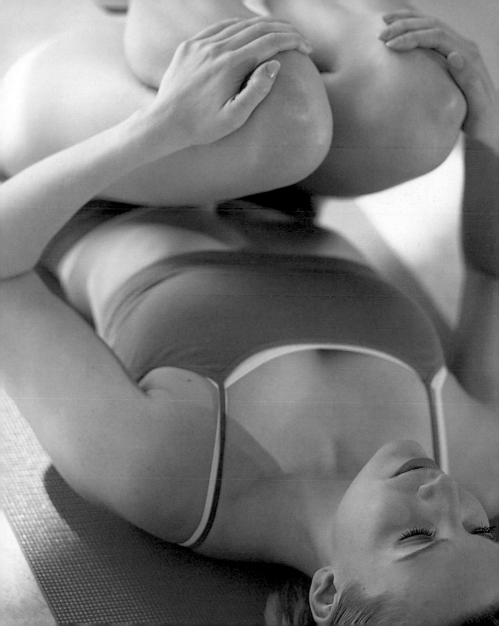

flexibility stretches

You may feel as though your muscles don't need stretching right now, but a few stretches will keep them long and lean. Do these moves in order. They should take only 5 minutes.

1 hip flexor
Kneel on both knees, then step forwards with one foot. Keep your other knee on the floor. Rest your hands on your front knee. Slide your back leg out behind you. Feel the stretch in your hip. Hold for 10–12 seconds. Repeat with your other leg.

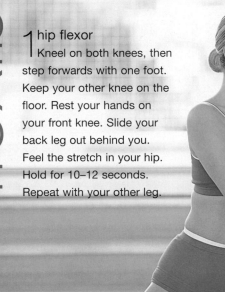

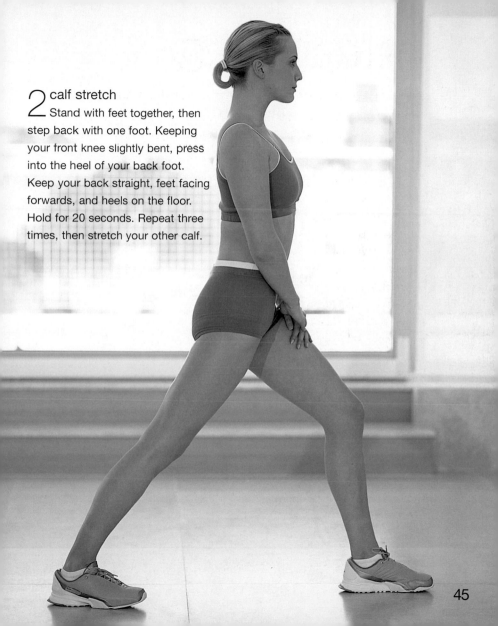

2 calf stretch

Stand with feet together, then step back with one foot. Keeping your front knee slightly bent, press into the heel of your back foot. Keep your back straight, feet facing forwards, and heels on the floor. Hold for 20 seconds. Repeat three times, then stretch your other calf.

3 lower back stretch

Lie on your back and hold the tops of your shins with both hands. Gently pull your knees in close to your body until you can feel the stretch in your lower back. Hold for 10 seconds, then slowly return to the start.

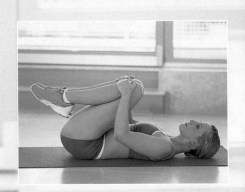

4 spine rotation

Still lying on your back, stretch your arms out at shoulder level. Bend both legs, then drop your knees to the side so one knee is touching the floor. Keep your shoulder blades flat on the floor, but don't force the stretch. Hold for 15 seconds, then slowly return to the start position. Repeat on your other side.

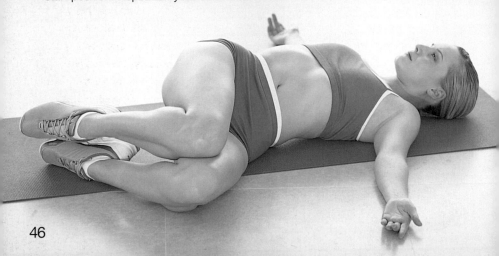

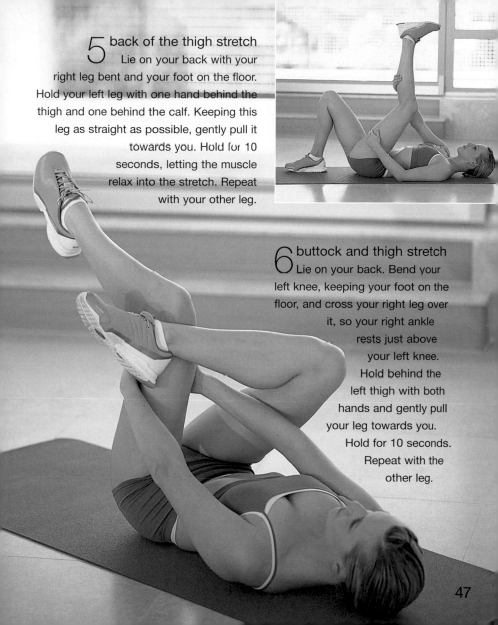

5 **back of the thigh stretch**
Lie on your back with your right leg bent and your foot on the floor. Hold your left leg with one hand behind the thigh and one behind the calf. Keeping this leg as straight as possible, gently pull it towards you. Hold for 10 seconds, letting the muscle relax into the stretch. Repeat with your other leg.

6 **buttock and thigh stretch**
Lie on your back. Bend your left knee, keeping your foot on the floor, and cross your right leg over it, so your right ankle rests just above your left knee. Hold behind the left thigh with both hands and gently pull your leg towards you. Hold for 10 seconds. Repeat with the other leg.

workout forum

I love working out on my own, but I also enjoy the motivation that comes from being in a group. Which classes are best for bums?

Try one of the many 'bums and tums' classes. These are a combination of regular aerobic exercise with floor work that's specifically designed to target your stomach and buttocks. They can be very effective. Body pump is another class that might fit the bill. Do bear in mind, though, that you shouldn't go overboard with this sort of class – the exercises work the muscles of the bottom so intensively that they can end up making it look a bit bulky.

I'm feeling much better about myself since I started doing the workouts and am inspired to improve my eating habits. What advice do you have?

That's great news. I often find that people go from strength to strength when they start tackling health and fitness issues and I'm always pleased to hear when my programmes have had a good effect on someone's self-image. In terms of food 'dos and don'ts', aim to eat a wide variety of foods, especially fruit, vegetables, and oily fish, so you get a good range of nutrients. Eat meat, wheat, and dairy products in moderation, and reduce or cut out tea, coffee, fizzy drinks, and alcohol. Use olive oil and sunflower oil, but avoid saturated fats (those that are solid at room temperature).

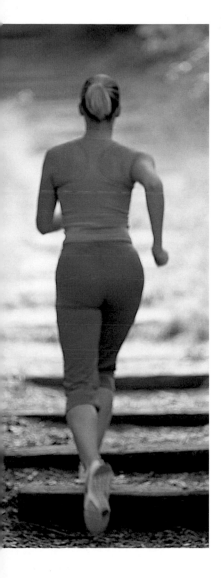

What kind of exercise can I do on my non-workout days?

Go for something low-impact, like front crawl swimming, hill-walking, or using the elliptical cross-trainer in the gym. About 30 minutes spent doing a moderate-intensity aerobic exercise like this will continue the toning work on the muscles of your bum and help maintain weight or promote fat loss. Make time to stretch for a few minutes at the end of every session. This keeps you flexible and wards off muscle aches and pains.

I drink lots of water while I'm exercising but I still felt thirsty at the end of the workout yesterday. I don't want to drink so much that I get a stitch, but how much should I drink?

To avoid a stitch, drink plenty of water before you even start exercising. Then, drink another two or three glasses while you're working out. Most of us are dehydrated a lot of the time. About 8 glasses (1.5–2 litres/2½–3½ pints) a day is the recommended amount. Aim for this, and get into the habit of drinking before you get thirsty – by then your body's already dehydrated anyway.

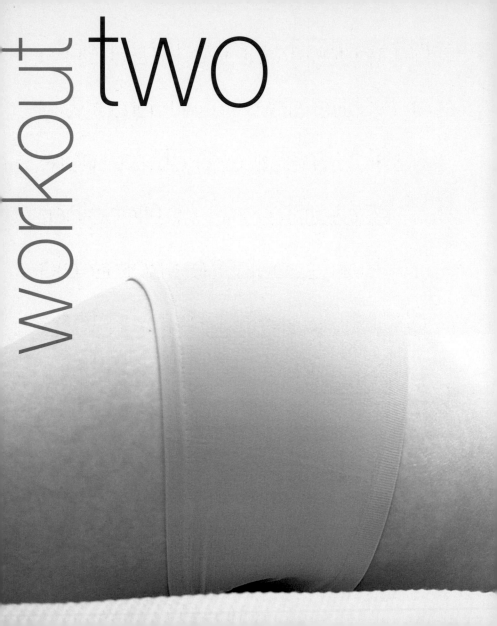

workout two

I'm taking your workload up a gear or two now. You'll probably find these exercises more explosive and challenging. You should see some big changes in your muscle tone too. Alternate this workout with the first one.

warm-up

To prime your muscles for the work to come, you need to warm up for 5–10 minutes, just as you did before workout one. If you chose to run at the last session, try power walking this time, and vice versa. Here are some more tips.

Power walking is great exercise for your buttocks. It makes them look lean and thin because you're using them as workhorses to power you forwards. Remember to:

- Keep your chin up and eyes ahead.
- Hold your tummy muscles tight.
- Keep your neck and shoulders relaxed.
- Avoid overstriding – keep your stride length short.

Running gets more enjoyable the more you do it. Make the most of it by:

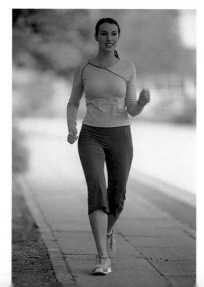

- Relaxing your shoulders.
- Using your arms to help your momentum: swing them forwards and backwards, but don't exaggerate the motion.
- Keeping your body upright and your tummy muscles pulled in tight.

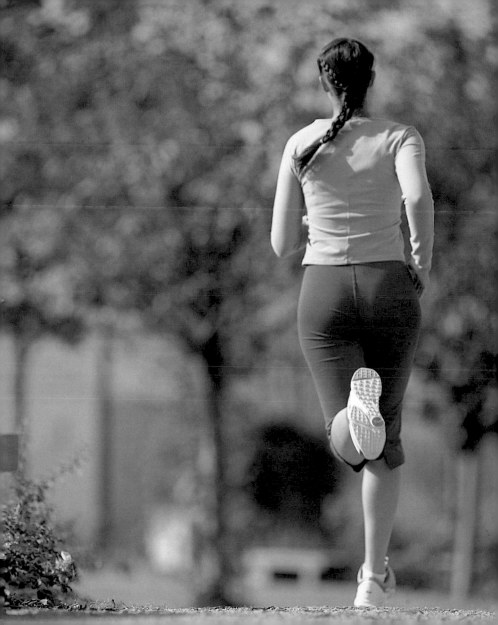

jump squat

An advanced squat that will test your legs completely. Let's see some air between your feet and the floor.

level ① do 15 squats

level ② do 25 squats

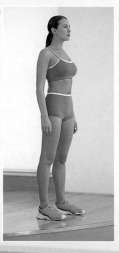

1 Stand with your feet hip-width apart, your back straight, and your arms relaxed by your sides. Bend your knees slightly, then jump up as high as possible.

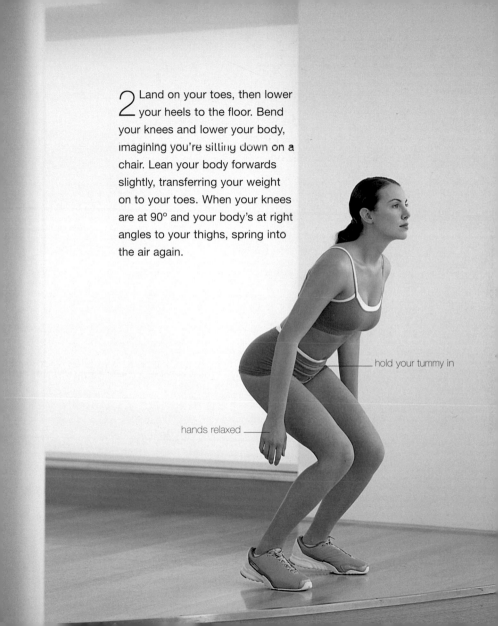

2 Land on your toes, then lower your heels to the floor. Bend your knees and lower your body, imagining you're sitting down on a chair. Lean your body forwards slightly, transferring your weight on to your toes. When your knees are at 90° and your body's at right angles to your thighs, spring into the air again.

hold your tummy in

hands relaxed

side bridge

This variation on the basic bridge works your obliques
hard and eradicates any trace of love handles.

level ① hold for 30 secs per side

level ② hold for 60 secs per side

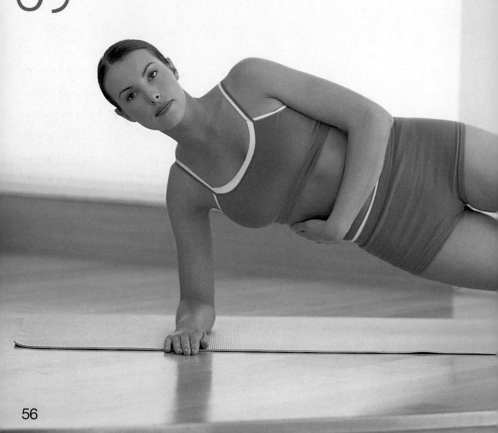

Lie on your side with one elbow and forearm directly under your shoulder as support. Place one foot on top of the other, then raise yourself up, keeping a straight line from your head to your toes. Use your oblique muscles to maintain the position and place one hand across your tummy to help you balance. Slowly return to the start, then repeat on the other side.

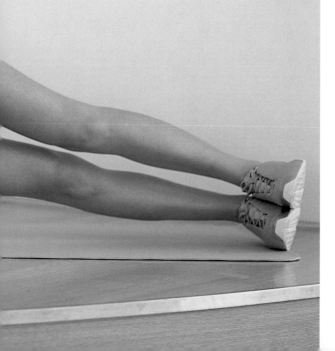

body talk

avoiding a bulky bum

A couple of sessions of your favourite aerobic activity every week should really trim your bottom. Or so you'd think. Some aerobic exercises actually work the muscles of your bottom so intensively that they can end up making it look bulky rather than toned. Step classes, step machines, cycling, and rollerblading all fall into this category. So go easy on them. If you have the chance, go hill walking, swim the front crawl, or use the elliptical cross-trainer in the gym instead.

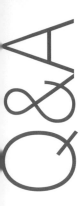

eating smart

My eating is fine and healthy all day, but goes to pieces in the evening, when I start raiding the freezer for tubs of ice cream and eating endless bits of toast. What can I do about it?

This is a fairly common scenario caused by one of two things. Check that you're eating enough earlier in the day. If you're not, your body's probably crying out for energy. It's then that a quick 'sugar fix' becomes unbearably tempting. Check too that you're not eating foods that are giving your body a quick supply of energy and then leaving it wanting more (there's more about this on page 37). Make sure you start each day with a hearty breakfast. Never be tempted to skip lunch, and have a 'strategic snack' in the middle of the afternoon to keep you going until dinner-time. Some vegetable sticks or a couple of pieces of orchard fruit are ideal.

I've heard about the 'golden half hour' after a workout when you can eat what you like and your body will burn it up. Is this true?

It's certainly true that your metabolism will be working more quickly for a few hours after exercise and that your body will be burning more calories as a result. But it's carbohydrates that your body needs then – like wholemeal bread, brown rice, wild rice, vegetables, pulses, and grains. So enjoy a sensible meal after your workout, rather than undoing all your hard work by eating or drinking high-calorie foods with little nutritional value.

What should I eat before and after a workout?

The best foods to go for – both before and after your session – are easily digested carbohydrates (*see left*). Beforehand they give you energy; afterwards they replace it. In an ideal world, you'll eat about 3 hours before you work out so that your stomach is empty. If this isn't always possible, do your utmost not to eat in the hour prior to exercising, as this can adversely affect your blood sugar levels.

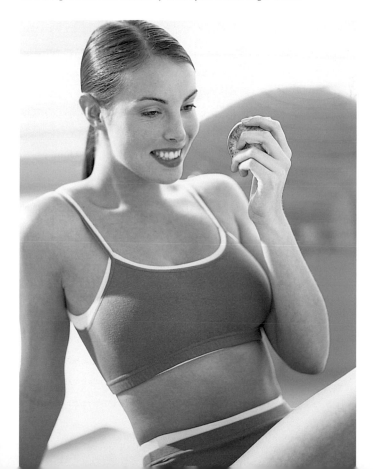

lunge

You may well need to clear yourself some space for this one.
Switch direction whenever you need to.

levels ① and ② do 20 lunges

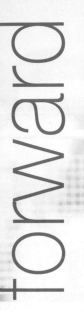

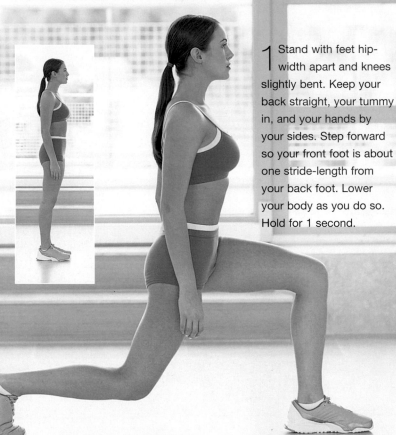

1 Stand with feet hip-width apart and knees slightly bent. Keep your back straight, your tummy in, and your hands by your sides. Step forward so your front foot is about one stride-length from your back foot. Lower your body as you do so. Hold for 1 second.

2 Raise your body, then step forward with your other leg. Lower your body as you did in step 1, then continue as before.

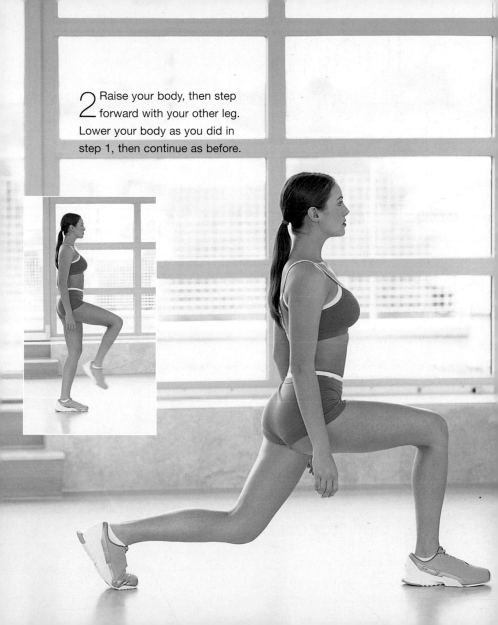

leg raise

It's really hard to balance on one foot (as you're about to find out), but it is extremely good for your waistline.

level ① hold for 20 secs per leg

level ② hold for 40 secs per leg

1 Position yourself with your toes on the floor and your elbows and forearms directly under your shoulders.

leg straight and in line with body

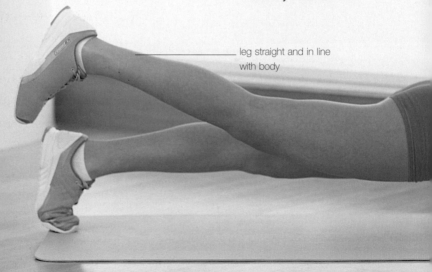

do it right

tummy muscles tight

The bridge leg raise works such wonders on your waistline, it's worth getting right. That said, it is tricky. If you're finding you wobble as soon as you raise your leg, double-check that you're squeezing your tummy muscles tight. This will really help you keep your balance. Reduce the distance you're raising your leg too. Start with just a tiny lift, then gradually build up to the full 30cm (12in) over the course of a few workouts.

2 Raise yourself up so you're supporting your body with your elbows, forearms, and toes. Keep a straight line from your shoulders to your ankles. Now raise one leg 15–30cm (6–12in). Hold the position still, squeezing your tummy muscles tight, for the required time. Slowly return to the start. Now switch legs and repeat.

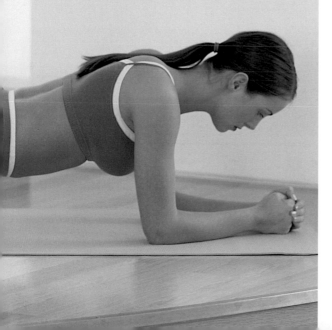

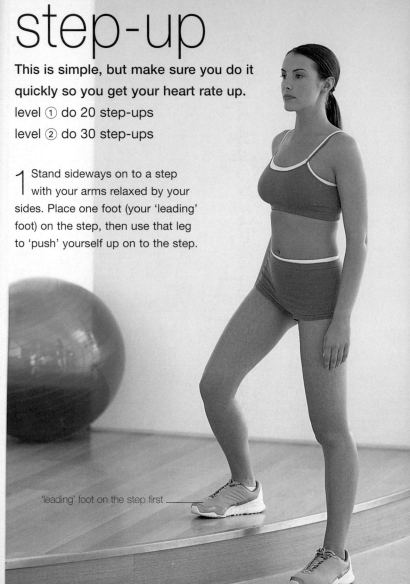

side step-up

This is simple, but make sure you do it quickly so you get your heart rate up.

level ① do 20 step-ups

level ② do 30 step-ups

1 Stand sideways on to a step with your arms relaxed by your sides. Place one foot (your 'leading' foot) on the step, then use that leg to 'push' yourself up on to the step.

'leading' foot on the step first

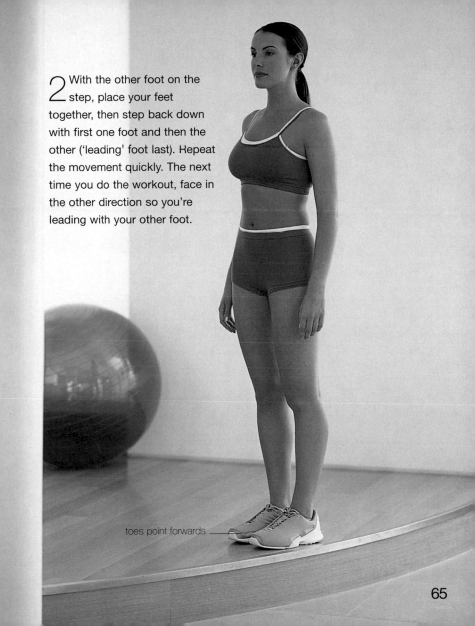

2 With the other foot on the step, place your feet together, then step back down with first one foot and then the other ('leading' foot last). Repeat the movement quickly. The next time you do the workout, face in the other direction so you're leading with your other foot.

toes point forwards

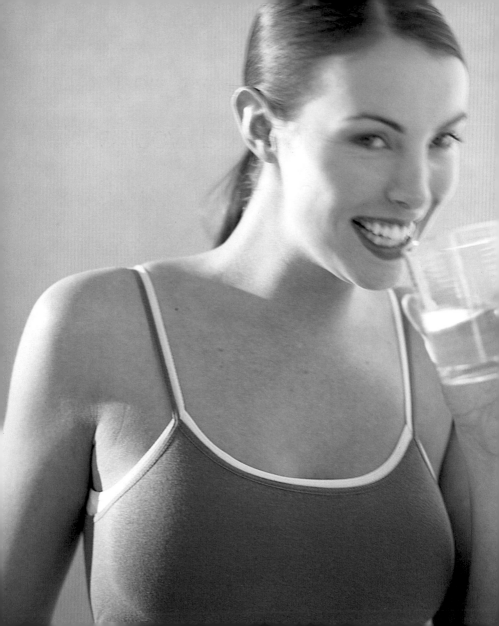

When you're working your muscles hard, your body needs water, no matter if you're sweating or not. Get into the habit of taking a sip every few minutes, and be prepared to get through half a litre or more during every workout.

side bridge raise

Watch you don't swing your hips about with this exercise. Concentrate on using your obliques and your hips to move your body in a controlled way.

level ① do 5–10 raises per side

level ② do 10–20 raises per side

1 Lie on your side with one elbow and forearm directly under your shoulder. Place one foot on top of the other, and position your other hand in front of you as support.

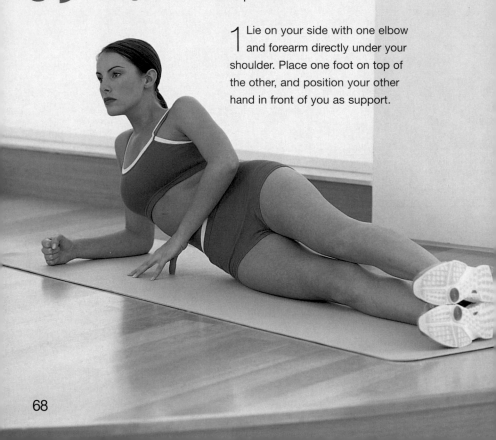

2 With the help of your supporting arm, raise your body, pushing your hips up as high as feels comfortable. Keep your body in a straight line – don't waver backwards or forwards. Slowly lower yourself to the start position. When you've done all the raises on one side, lie on your other side and repeat the exercise.

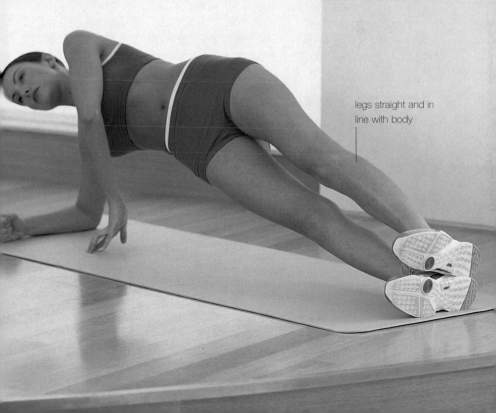

legs straight and in
line with body

reverse curl crunch

A nice variation on the classic sit-up, but raising your legs like this brings the muscles of your lower abdomen into play early on in the movement. As a result, the exercise is intensive from the word 'go'.

level ① do 15 crunches
level ② do 30 crunches

1 Lie on your back with your hands by your ears. Raise your legs in the air, soles of your feet facing upwards. Keep a slight bend in your knees so your tummy muscles tighten.

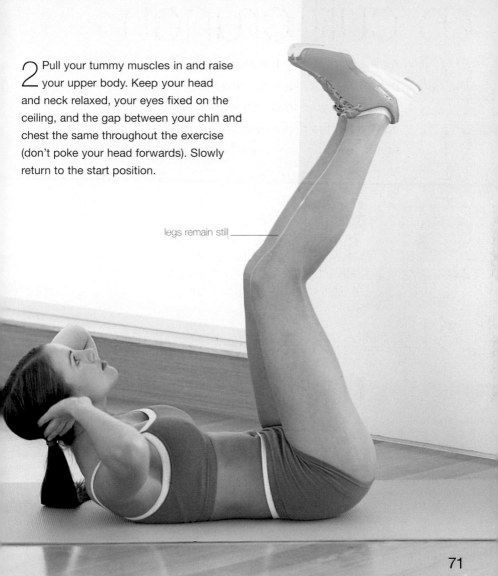

2 Pull your tummy muscles in and raise your upper body. Keep your head and neck relaxed, your eyes fixed on the ceiling, and the gap between your chin and chest the same throughout the exercise (don't poke your head forwards). Slowly return to the start position.

legs remain still

power lunge

Power's the operative word here. A powerful 'spring back' in step 2 recruits a large number of muscle groups and creates strong, lean legs.

level ① do 15 lunges per leg

level ② do 30 lunges per leg

stand tall, tummy pulled in

1 Stand with your feet together and your hands relaxed by your sides. Tuck your chin in and look straight ahead.

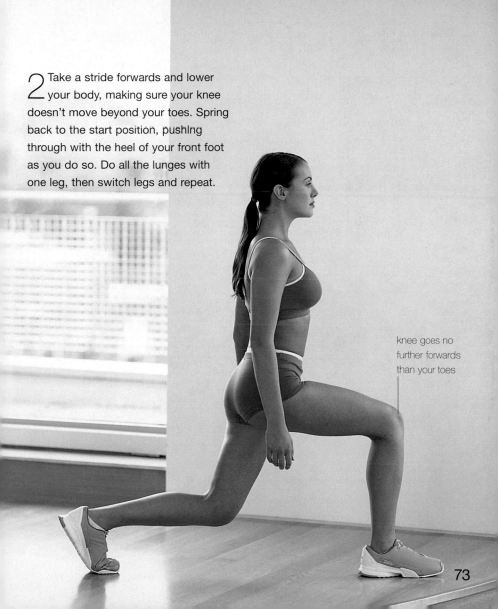

2 Take a stride forwards and lower your body, making sure your knee doesn't move beyond your toes. Spring back to the start position, pushing through with the heel of your front foot as you do so. Do all the lunges with one leg, then switch legs and repeat.

knee goes no further forwards than your toes

73

tummy talk

My posture's improved since I started exercising, but I'm still aware of slumping at my desk in the office. How can I keep my tummy working when I spend all day sitting down?

Here's an exercise you can do in the office every time you think of it. It will make you sit up straight and stop your 'innards' pushing your tummy muscles forward and stretching them. Gently pull your stomach muscles in as if you were trying to make your belly button press against your spine. At the same time, tuck your chin in and imagine a string pulling the top of your head up to the ceiling. Pull your shoulders back and relax them.

My tummy's now flat, but it still wobbles a bit if I run or jump. Is this something I have to live with or can I firm it up?

To reduce the fat on your tummy, you'll need to reduce your total body fat level by exercise and a healthy diet. How successful you'll be depends ultimately on your body shape: if you're apple-shaped, you'll naturally carry more fat around your tummy; if you're pear-shaped, on the other hand, you'll carry any excess around your hips and thighs. Either way, you'll look and feel better with the minimum amount of body fat.

I'm sleeping much more soundly since I started exercising. Why is that?

Many jobs today are sedentary and computer-based, so by night-time your brain is overtired and your body's underused – hardly a recipe for a good night's sleep. Exercise redresses the balance by easing tension in your muscles and relaxing you generally. Apart from sleeping better, you may well have noticed some other benefits too. As well as improved digestion and circulation, your mood should be better since exercise stimulates your brain to release endorphins, its natural 'feel-good' chemicals.

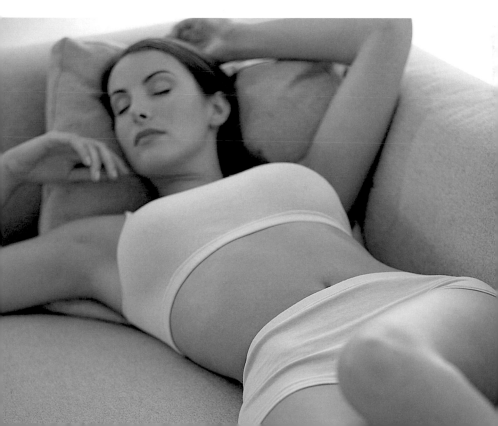

oblique

Raising your legs in the air for this exercise means you use your abdominal muscles to keep your balance. Make sure you keep your legs still to maximize the exercise's effectiveness.

level ① do 20 obliques

level ② do 40 obliques

1 Lie on your back with your knees together and your thighs at 90° to the floor. Keep your tummy muscles pulled in tight and your back pressed into the floor. Place your hands by your ears.

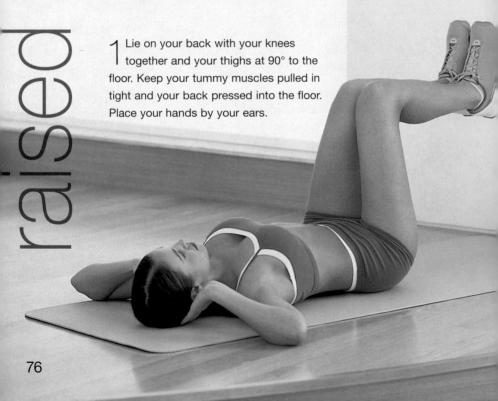

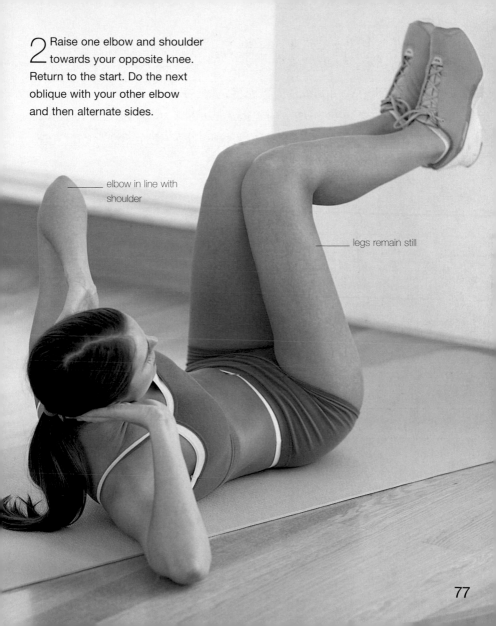

2 Raise one elbow and shoulder towards your opposite knee. Return to the start. Do the next oblique with your other elbow and then alternate sides.

_____ elbow in line with shoulder

_____ legs remain still

glute raise

This lifts your bottom and gives the muscles in your buttocks (glutes) a firmer, more pert appearance. To maximize the lifting effect, make sure you push up into the heel and hold your tummy muscles tight.

level ① do 30 raises per leg

level ② do 40 raises per leg

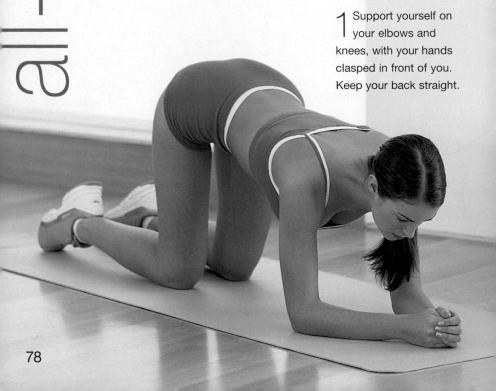

1 Support yourself on your elbows and knees, with your hands clasped in front of you. Keep your back straight.

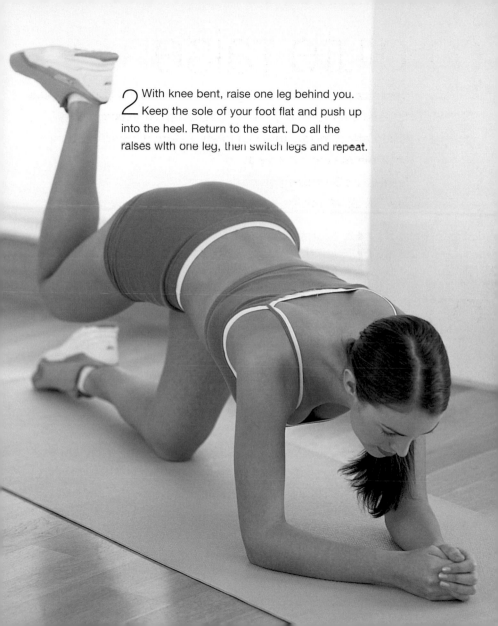

2 With knee bent, raise one leg behind you. Keep the sole of your foot flat and push up into the heel. Return to the start. Do all the raises with one leg, then switch legs and repeat.

oblique knee pull-in

The closer you can get your elbow and shoulder to your knee, the more you'll work your waistline. Focus on the quality of the movement, but make sure you lift your shoulder too.

level ① do 15 pull-ins per side

level ② do 25 pull-ins per side

1 Lie on your back with one foot flat on the floor and the other leg raised so your thigh is at right angles to the floor. Place your hands by your ears and keep your shoulders down.

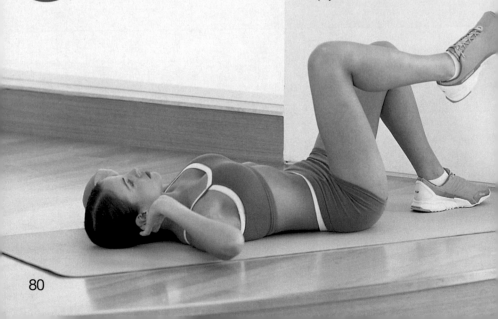

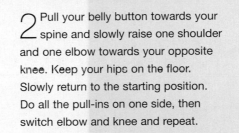

2 Pull your belly button towards your spine and slowly raise one shoulder and one elbow towards your opposite knee. Keep your hips on the floor. Slowly return to the starting position. Do all the pull-ins on one side, then switch elbow and knee and repeat.

elbow in line
with shoulder

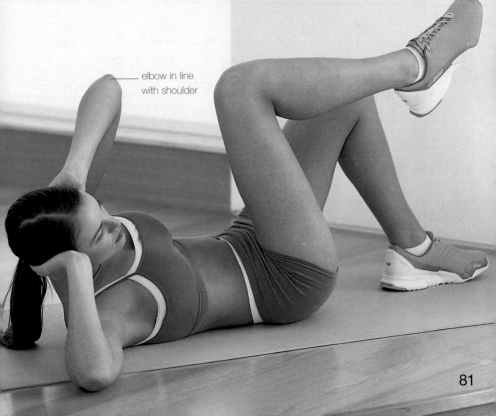

In many ways, these workouts are about creating your body's own 'corset'. The harder you work, the tighter you pull the strings. But unlike the whale-bone contraption your granny once wore, a natural corset's there the whole time, making you look fantastic 24/7.

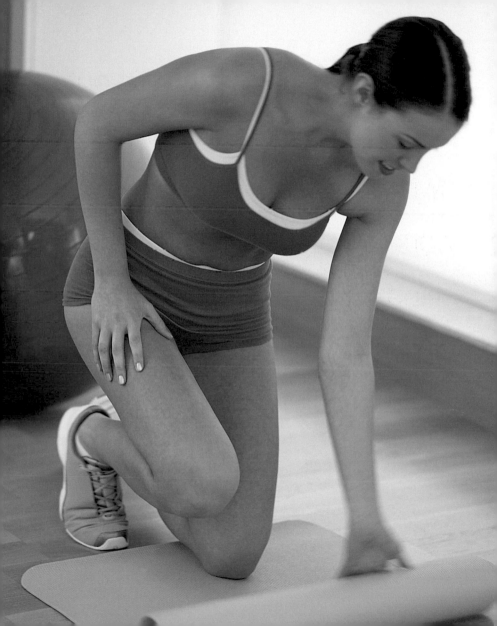

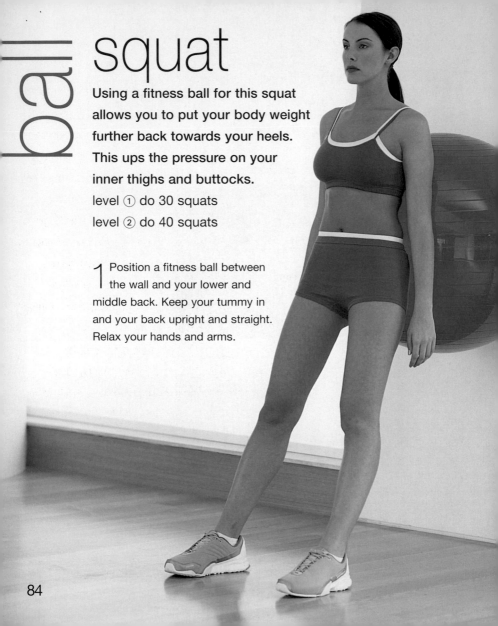

squat

Using a fitness ball for this squat allows you to put your body weight further back towards your heels. This ups the pressure on your inner thighs and buttocks.

level ① do 30 squats

level ② do 40 squats

1 Position a fitness ball between the wall and your lower and middle back. Keep your tummy in and your back upright and straight. Relax your hands and arms.

2 Slowly lower your body until your thighs are parallel with the floor. Slowly push yourself back to the start.

repeat the workout
When you've done all the squats, go back to the beginning (page 54) and do all the exercises again in order. When you've done the ball squat again, finish workout two with the stretch moves overleaf.

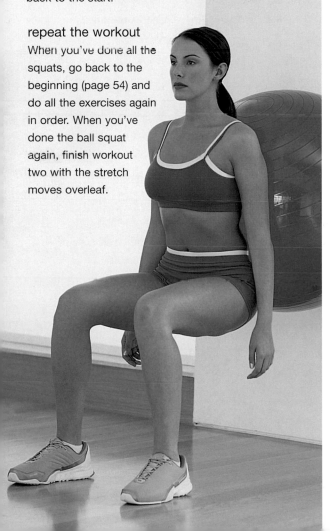

variation

avoiding the shakes
This is the last exercise in this workout. When you come to do it for the second time, your muscles will be starting to tire. If you find it too much of a strain and your legs begin to wobble, walk round the room and shake your legs out before going on to the stretching sequence overleaf.

making it easier
If you find the ball squat altogether too difficult, lower yourself down a little less. With practice, you should be able to lower yourself more and more each time.

stretches

Finish workout two in the same way you rounded off workout one – with a sequence of stretches. They'll eliminate tension, improve suppleness, and reduce the chance of soreness.

1 hip flexor

Kneel on both knees, then step forwards with one foot. Keep your other knee on the floor. Rest your hands on your front knee. Slide your back leg out behind you. Feel the stretch in your hip. Hold for 10–12 seconds. Repeat with your other leg.

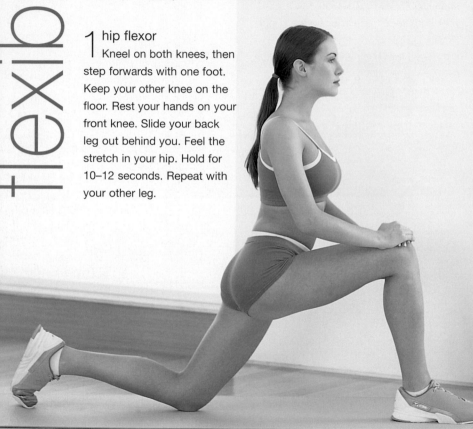

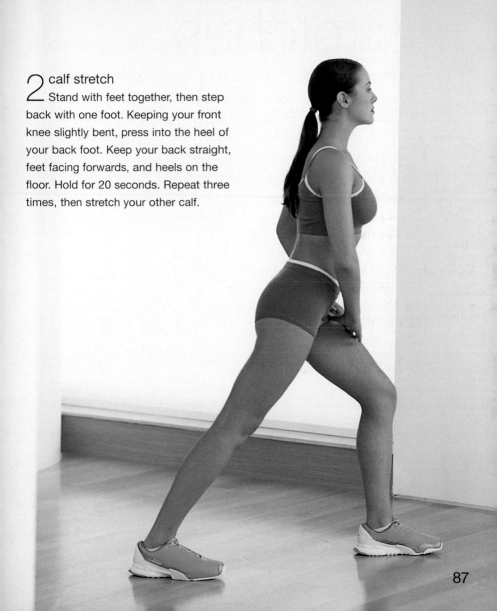

2 calf stretch

Stand with feet together, then step back with one foot. Keeping your front knee slightly bent, press into the heel of your back foot. Keep your back straight, feet facing forwards, and heels on the floor. Hold for 20 seconds. Repeat three times, then stretch your other calf.

87

3 lower back stretch

Lie on your back and hold the tops of your shins with both hands. Gently pull your knees in close to your body until you can feel the stretch in your lower back. Hold for 10 seconds, then slowly return to the start.

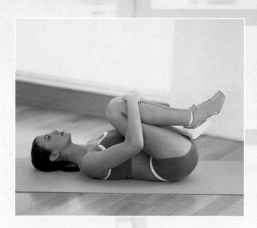

4 spine rotation

Still lying on your back, stretch your arms out at shoulder level. Bend both legs, then drop your knees to the side so one knee is touching the floor. Keep your shoulder blades flat on the floor, but don't force the stretch. Hold for 15 seconds, then slowly return to the start position. Repeat on your other side.

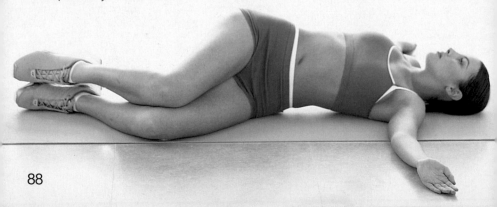

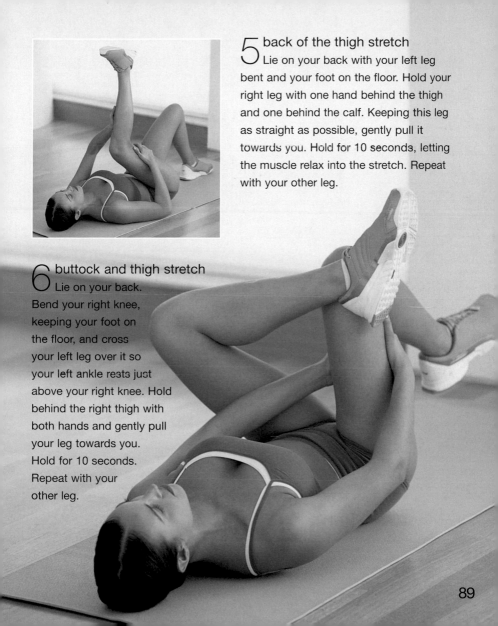

5 back of the thigh stretch
Lie on your back with your left leg bent and your foot on the floor. Hold your right leg with one hand behind the thigh and one behind the calf. Keeping this leg as straight as possible, gently pull it towards you. Hold for 10 seconds, letting the muscle relax into the stretch. Repeat with your other leg.

6 buttock and thigh stretch
Lie on your back. Bend your right knee, keeping your foot on the floor, and cross your left leg over it so your left ankle rests just above your right knee. Hold behind the right thigh with both hands and gently pull your leg towards you. Hold for 10 seconds. Repeat with your other leg.

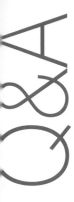

keeping it up

How can I keep my tummy flat now I've got it flat?

Well, you'll be delighted to hear that it's far easier to 'maintain' a flat tummy than it is to get one in the first place. Keep an eye on the level you're working at. If you started at level ①, upgrade to level ②. If you're already at level ②, repeat each workout twice (ie do them three times all the way through) rather than just once. Check too that you do the exercises correctly – sloppy work makes for a sloppy body.

Will my bum get bigger if I carry on exercising?

Only if you take up a weights programme or do loads of step classes. If you carry on at the same level as I recommended at the beginning of the book (exercising every other day), you'll be doing pretty much the right amount of exercise to maintain the great muscle tone you've gained, but at no risk of bulking up. Moderation does it!

How can I vary my workout routine?

Think about changing the way you warm up for a start. Instead of running or walking, try cycling or going for a swim. You might want to think about asking a friend if she'd like to exercise alongside you – a training buddy is brilliant for keeping you motivated (and for chivvying you when your enthusiasm starts to flag). If your budget will stretch to it, you could do worse than hire a personal trainer of course!

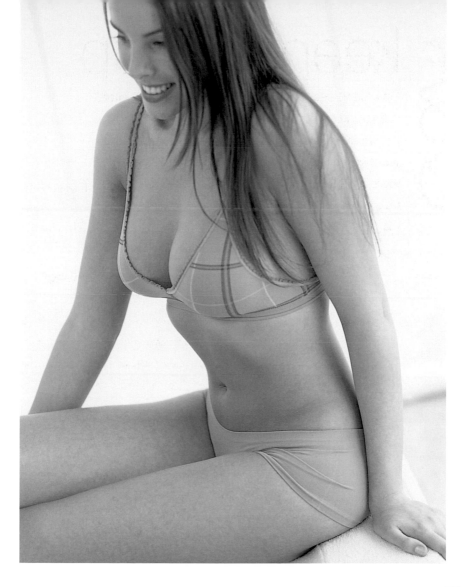

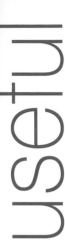

information

which fitness level?

Before you start the workouts, you need to know your fitness level – ① or ②.
If you're currently taking little or no exercise, start at level ①. If you already do
30 minutes or more aerobic exercise (that's enough to make you puff and
sweat) three times a week, start at level ②. If you're a level ① user and you
start to find the routines too easy, upgrade yourself to level ②. Similarly, level
② users who start to find the routines a cinch should do each workout three
times all the way through rather than just twice.

how often to peform the workouts

Aim to perform each workout twice a week. Do them alternately.

the equipment you need

I've designed these workouts for you to do at home, so they're ideal
performed on a hardwood floor or carpet. If you're at all concerned that you
might slip, however, think about investing in a non-slip exercise mat or yoga
mat like the ones we've used in this book (the address of the supplier is listed
on the last page). The only piece of equipment you absolutely need is a fitness
ball. You'll sometimes see these called Swiss balls, stability balls, gym balls,
back balls, or birth balls. I think they're great: they make exercise fun and
improve your balance as well as toning your muscles. They come in three
sizes according to your height and weight. The medium size is correct for

most women (though you may prefer the small size if you're under 1.55m/5ft 2in). You can buy them from most sports shops and department stores, but in case you have any problems tracking them down I've given you some suppliers below.

suppliers of fitness balls

If you can't find fitness balls in your local shops, you can order them from the following suppliers:

In the UK
Physique Management
0870 60 70 381
www.physique.co.uk

In Australia
www.simplefitnesssolutions.com

In New Zealand
www.fitnessworks.co.nz

index

A

aerobic exercise *49*
aerobic warm-up *12, 52*
all-fours glute raise *78–9*
apple-shaped body *74*

B

back, lower back stretch *46, 88*
balls *see* fitness balls
bloating *36*
blood sugar levels *37, 59*
body raise on ball *26–7*
breathing *15*
bridge: basic bridge *40–1*
  bridge leg raise *62–3*
  side bridge *56–7*
  side bridge raise *68–9*
bulking up *57, 90*
buttocks: buttock and thigh stretch *47, 89*
  glute raises *16–17, 78–9*
  resistance work *20*

C

calf stretch *45, 87*
calories *36, 58*
carbohydrates *58, 59*
cellulite *41*
classes *48*
core strength *20*
cross-trainer *49, 57*
crunches: extended leg crunch *30–1*
  full crunch *18–19*
  reverse curl crunch *70–1*
curls: hamstrings curl with ball *22–3*
  reverse curl crunch *70–1*

reverse curl with ball *24–5*
cycling *90*

D

dehydration *15, 49*
detoxing *41*
diet *48, 58–9*
  weight loss *21, 36*
  wheat intolerance *36*

E

endorphins *75*
extended leg crunch *30–1*

F

fat: cellulite *41*
  on tummy *74*
fitness balls *92–3*
  ball oblique *34–5*
  ball squat *84–5*
  body raise on ball *26–7*
  hamstrings curl with ball *22–3*
  reverse curl with ball *24–5*
forward lunge *60–1*
full crunch *18–19*

G

glute raise: all-fours *78–9*
  prone *16–17*

H

hamstrings curl with ball *22–3*
heart rate *32, 64*
hip flexor stretch *44, 86*

J
jump squat *54–5*

K
knee pull-in, oblique *80–1*
knee raise *33*

L
leg raise, bridge *62–3*
lunges: forward lunge *60–1*
  simple lunge *38–9*

M
metabolic rate *58*

O
oblique muscles: ball oblique *34–5*
  oblique knee pull-in *80–1*
  raised knee oblique *76–7*

P
pear-shaped body *20, 74*
posture *74*
power walking *12, 52*
prone glute raise *16–17*

R
raised knee oblique *76–7*
resistance work *20*
rests (between exercises) *15*
reverse curl crunch *70–1*
reverse curl with ball *24–5*
running *12, 20, 52*

S
seated squat *14–15*
shakes, avoiding *85*
side bridge *56–7*
side bridge raise *68–9*

side step-up *64–5*
sleep *75*
snacks *58*
spine rotation *46, 88*
squats: ball squat *84–5*
  jump squat *54–5*
  seated squat *14–15*
step machines *57*
step-ups: knee raise *33*
  side step-up *64–5*
  simple step-up *32–3*
stitch, avoiding *49*
stretches *44–7, 86–9*
  back of the thigh *47, 89*
  buttock and thigh *47, 89*
  calf *45, 87*
  hip flexor *44, 86*
  lower back *46, 88*
  spine rotation *46, 88*
sugar *37, 58*
swimming *49, 57, 90*

W
waist exercises *20*
walking *12, 19, 52, 57*
warm-up *12, 52*
water, drinking *15, 49, 67*
weight loss *21, 36*
wheat intolerance *36*

author's credits

Thanks to everybody (too many of you to name, alas) who helped me with this book. A special thank you to the DK team, to Michael, Tracy, and Anna, in particular; to Russell for the great shots; to my own team, especially Nik, Richard, Jason, Ayo, and Alan; and to my brother Jon, who, as always, shared the workload with me. For more information about Matt Roberts Personal Training, please contact:

matt roberts personal training
32–34 Jermyn St
London SW1Y 6HS
Tel: 020 7439 8800
www.personaltrainer.uk.com

publisher's credits

Thanks to our models Janine Newberry and Kirsty Spence from ModelPlan, and to Nessie at ModelPlan; to Matt's team of trainers: Nik Cook, George Dick, Jason Hughes, Ayo Williams, and Alan Foley; to Toko at Hers and to Cor Kwakernaak for hair and make-up; to stylist Jo Atkins-Hughes; and to photography assistant Nina Duncan. Many thanks to Reebok for the kind loan of trainers for this book (all enquiries 0800 30 50 50) and to Agoy for the kind loan of the exercise mats (all enquiries 0208 933 8421 or at www.agoy.com).

about the author

Matt Roberts, the UK's hottest personal trainer, began as an international sprinter. He went on to complete his studies at the American Council for Exercise and the American College of Sports Medicine. Affectionately known as 'the personal trainer to the stars', Matt has an enviable reputation for training celebrities, among them Sandra Bullock, Trudie Styler, Mel C, Natalie Imbruglia, Naomi Campbell, Tom Ford, John Galliano, and Faye Dunaway. Alongside this high-profile client list, Matt derives equal satisfaction from helping each of his clients meet their health and fitness goals. And in his quest to make fitness and good health accessible to everyone, he produces his own range of vitamins, home gym equipment, and body care products.